The Healing Power of Yoga: Nurturing Mental Health for All

Alice Johansson

Copyright © [2023]

Author: Alice Johansson

Title: The Healing Power of Yoga: Nurturing Mental Health for All

This book is a product of [Publisher's Alice Johansson]

ISBN:

TABLE OF CONTENTS

Chapter 1: The Basics of Yoga and Mental Health

Understanding Yoga and its Benefits

Yoga is a practice that has been around for thousands of years and has gained immense popularity in recent times. It is not just a physical exercise but a holistic approach towards achieving mental, emotional, and spiritual well-being. In this subchapter, we will delve into the essence of yoga and explore its myriad benefits for individuals from all walks of life.

At its core, yoga is a discipline that combines physical postures (asanas), breathing techniques (pranayama), and meditation to create a union between the body, mind, and soul. It originated in ancient India and has since spread across the globe, captivating people of all ages and backgrounds. What sets yoga apart from other forms of exercise is its emphasis on mindfulness and self-awareness. Through the practice of yoga, individuals are encouraged to be fully present in the moment, fostering a deep connection with themselves and the world around them.

The benefits of yoga are far-reaching, extending beyond the physical realm. Regular practice can enhance flexibility, strength, and balance, but it also promotes relaxation, stress reduction, and mental clarity. Yoga has been shown to alleviate symptoms of anxiety and depression, improve sleep quality, boost self-esteem, and enhance overall mental health. By cultivating a sense of inner peace and tranquility, it empowers individuals to cope with the challenges of everyday life and find harmony amidst chaos.

Furthermore, yoga is a versatile practice that can be tailored to suit individual needs and preferences. Whether you are a beginner or an experienced yogi, there are various styles and levels of intensity to choose from. From gentle, restorative yoga to more vigorous practices like power yoga or hot yoga, there is something for everyone. Additionally, yoga can be practiced in a group setting or in the comfort of your own home, making it accessible to individuals with diverse lifestyles and schedules.

In conclusion, yoga is a powerful tool for self-transformation and personal growth. Its numerous benefits extend beyond the physical realm, nurturing mental health and well-being for all who embrace it. Regardless of your age, fitness level, or background, yoga offers a pathway to self-discovery, inner peace, and a more balanced life. So, take a deep breath, roll out your mat, and embark on a journey of healing and self-exploration through the transformative practice of yoga.

The Connection between Yoga and Mental Health

Yoga, an ancient practice originating from India, has gained immense popularity worldwide in recent years. While its physical benefits are widely acknowledged, the connection between yoga and mental health is often overlooked. In this subchapter, we will explore the profound impact yoga can have on nurturing mental health for all.

Yoga is not just a physical exercise; it is a holistic practice that encompasses the mind, body, and spirit. It incorporates various techniques such as postures (asanas), breathing exercises (pranayama), and meditation (dhyana) to bring about a state of balance and harmony within oneself. These practices have been proven to have a direct influence on mental well-being.

One of the primary ways yoga promotes mental health is through stress reduction. In today's fast-paced and demanding world, stress has become a common factor contributing to mental health issues such as anxiety and depression. Yoga helps individuals manage stress by activating the parasympathetic nervous system, which induces a relaxation response in the body. This, in turn, reduces the production of stress hormones and promotes a sense of calmness and tranquility.

Moreover, yoga encourages mindfulness and self-awareness. Through regular practice, individuals learn to observe their thoughts, emotions, and bodily sensations without judgment. This heightened awareness allows them to identify and address negative patterns of thinking and behavior, leading to improved mental clarity and emotional stability.

Additionally, yoga enhances the connection between the mind and body. Many mental health issues manifest as physical symptoms, and vice versa. By practicing yoga, individuals develop a deeper understanding of their bodies and learn to listen to its signals. This mind-body connection enables them to recognize and address the underlying causes of their mental health concerns, leading to a more holistic approach to healing.

Furthermore, yoga fosters a sense of community and social support. Attending yoga classes or joining yoga communities allows individuals to connect with like-minded individuals and build meaningful relationships. The support and camaraderie experienced in these settings can greatly contribute to one's mental well-being, reducing feelings of isolation and loneliness.

In conclusion, the connection between yoga and mental health is undeniable. Incorporating yoga into one's daily routine can have a transformative effect on mental well-being, promoting stress reduction, mindfulness, self-awareness, and a sense of community. Whether you are a yoga enthusiast or someone new to the practice, embracing yoga as a tool for nurturing mental health is beneficial for everyone.

Chapter 2: Yoga Poses and Techniques for Mental Wellness

Gentle Yoga Poses for Stress Relief

In today's fast-paced world, stress has become an inevitable part of our lives. From demanding work schedules to personal responsibilities, it's easy to feel overwhelmed and anxious. Fortunately, yoga offers a powerful solution for managing stress and finding inner calm. In this subchapter, we will explore a variety of gentle yoga poses specifically designed to relieve stress and promote mental well-being.

Yoga, an ancient practice originating from India, combines physical postures, breathing exercises, and meditation to enhance overall health and balance the mind, body, and spirit. It is a versatile practice that can be adapted to suit people of all ages and fitness levels. Gentle yoga, in particular, focuses on slow, deliberate movements and emphasizes relaxation and mindfulness.

One of the most effective poses for stress relief is the Child's Pose. This posture involves sitting on your knees and gently lowering your upper body to the ground, with your arms extended in front of you. This simple pose helps to release tension in the back, shoulders, and neck, while also promoting deep breathing and relaxation.

Another great pose for stress relief is the Legs-Up-The-Wall pose. This pose involves lying on your back with your legs extended vertically against a wall. This gentle inversion helps to calm the nervous system, increase blood circulation, and reduce anxiety and fatigue.

The Corpse Pose, or Savasana, is a classic yoga pose that is often practiced at the end of a yoga session. It involves lying flat on your back with your arms and legs relaxed, allowing your body to completely let go and enter a state of deep relaxation. Savasana is a powerful tool for stress relief as it helps to reduce muscle tension, lower blood pressure, and quiet the mind.

In addition to these poses, practicing gentle yoga regularly can also have a profound impact on your overall mental health. By incorporating deep breathing exercises and mindfulness techniques into your practice, you can cultivate a sense of inner peace and develop the skills to manage stress more effectively in your daily life.

Remember, yoga is a journey, and it's important to listen to your body and honor its limitations. If you're new to yoga or have any physical concerns, it's always best to consult with a qualified yoga instructor or healthcare professional before starting a new practice.

So, take a moment to breathe deeply, roll out your mat, and embark on a journey of stress relief through gentle yoga. Your mind, body, and spirit will thank you. Namaste.

Restorative Yoga for Relaxation and Anxiety Reduction

In today's fast-paced world, finding moments of peace and tranquility can seem like an impossible task. The constant demands of work, family, and social obligations can leave us feeling overwhelmed, stressed, and anxious. Thankfully, restorative yoga offers a powerful solution to these modern-day challenges. By incorporating this gentle and nurturing practice into our lives, we can experience deep relaxation, reduce anxiety, and cultivate a sense of overall well-being.

Restorative yoga is a passive form of yoga that focuses on relaxation and healing. It involves holding gentle poses for an extended period, usually supported by props such as blankets, bolsters, and blocks. This support allows the body to fully relax, releasing tension and promoting a sense of deep calmness. As we settle into each pose, the mind can gradually quiet down, allowing us to let go of negative thoughts and worries.

One of the key benefits of restorative yoga is its ability to reduce anxiety. By engaging in slow, mindful movements and deep, conscious breathing, we activate the body's relaxation response, also known as the parasympathetic nervous system. This response counteracts the fight-or-flight response that often dominates our lives and contributes to feelings of anxiety. As the body relaxes, the mind follows suit, helping to alleviate stress and promote a sense of inner peace.

Furthermore, restorative yoga offers a unique opportunity for self-care and self-compassion. In a society that glorifies busyness and productivity, taking the time to slow down and nurture ourselves can feel indulgent or even selfish. However, by prioritizing our mental and emotional well-being, we become better equipped to handle life's challenges and responsibilities. Restorative yoga allows us to show ourselves kindness and compassion, fostering a deeper connection with our bodies, minds, and spirits.

Whether you are an experienced yogi or new to the practice, restorative yoga can be a valuable addition to your self-care routine. It is accessible to people of all ages and fitness levels, making it an inclusive practice that can benefit everyone. By dedicating just a few minutes a day to restorative yoga, you can experience the transformative power of relaxation, reduce anxiety, and cultivate a greater sense of overall well-being.

So, carve out a little space in your day, roll out your mat, and allow yourself to be enveloped in the soothing embrace of restorative yoga. Your mind, body, and spirit will thank you.

Yoga Breathing Exercises for Improved Mental Clarity

In today's fast-paced world, it is not uncommon for our minds to feel overwhelmed and cluttered. We often find ourselves struggling to focus, experiencing mental fog, and feeling disconnected from our true selves. Fortunately, the ancient practice of yoga offers a powerful solution to these modern-day challenges – breathing exercises.

Yoga breathing exercises, also known as pranayama, can have a profound impact on our mental clarity and overall well-being. By incorporating these simple yet effective techniques into our daily lives, we can cultivate a calm and focused mind, leading to improved mental health and enhanced productivity.

One such technique is the "Ujjayi" breath, which translates to "victorious breath." This deep, audible breath involves a slight constriction of the throat, creating a gentle hissing sound. By practicing Ujjayi breath, we can slow down our breath and regulate our energy, bringing a sense of calm and clarity to our minds.

Another beneficial breathing exercise is "Nadi Shodhana," or alternate nostril breathing. This technique helps balance the left and right sides of the brain, promoting mental harmony and improved concentration. By using the thumb and ring finger to alternate between blocking the nostrils, we can create a harmonizing effect on our mental and emotional states.

Additionally, "Kapalabhati" breath, or skull-shining breath, is an invigorating technique that energizes the body and clears the mind. This rapid, forceful exhalation followed by a passive inhalation helps release stagnant energy and toxins, leaving us feeling refreshed and mentally alert.

Practicing these breathing exercises regularly can bring about a multitude of benefits. Not only do they help calm the mind and reduce stress, but they also enhance our ability to focus and make clearer decisions. By oxygenating the brain and improving circulation, these exercises improve mental clarity, memory, and overall cognitive function.

Whether you are a seasoned yogi or a beginner exploring the world of yoga, incorporating these breathing practices into your daily routine can have a profound impact on your mental well-being. So, take a moment each day to connect with your breath, to find stillness within, and to nurture your mental health. Embrace the healing power of yoga and experience the transformative effects of these simple yet potent breathing exercises.

Meditation and Mindfulness Practices for Mental Stability

In today's fast-paced and stressful world, mental stability is a precious commodity that many of us seek. The good news is that within the realm of yoga, there exists a powerful tool that can help us find the calm and tranquility we so desperately crave. This tool is none other than meditation and mindfulness practices.

Meditation has been practiced for thousands of years and is a cornerstone of yoga. It involves training the mind to focus and redirect our thoughts, ultimately leading to a state of mental clarity and stability. By quieting the mind and allowing ourselves to be fully present in the moment, we can cultivate a sense of inner peace and balance.

Mindfulness, on the other hand, is about being fully aware of our thoughts, feelings, and bodily sensations in the present moment. It is a practice that encourages us to observe these experiences without judgment or attachment. By practicing mindfulness, we can develop a deeper understanding of ourselves and our emotions, which in turn can lead to enhanced mental stability.

Both meditation and mindfulness can offer numerous benefits for our mental health. Research has shown that regular meditation practice can reduce stress, anxiety, and depression. It can also improve focus, attention, and overall cognitive function. Similarly, mindfulness practices have been found to increase self-awareness and self-compassion, reduce rumination, and improve overall psychological well-being.

To incorporate these practices into your daily life, start by setting aside a dedicated time and space for meditation. Find a quiet and comfortable spot where you can sit or lie down without distractions. Begin by focusing on your breath, observing its natural rhythm without trying to change it. As thoughts arise, acknowledge them without judgment and gently bring your attention back to your breath.

For mindfulness, aim to bring a sense of awareness to your daily activities. Whether you're eating, walking, or even brushing your teeth, try to fully engage your senses and be present in the moment. Notice the taste, texture, and smell of your food, feel the sensation of your feet touching the ground as you walk, or observe the bristles of your toothbrush against your teeth.

Remember, both meditation and mindfulness are practices that require patience and consistency. Start with just a few minutes each day and gradually increase the duration as you become more comfortable. Over time, you will begin to experience the profound benefits of these practices and witness the transformative power they can have on your mental stability.

In conclusion, meditation and mindfulness practices are invaluable tools that can help us achieve and maintain mental stability in our fast-paced world. By incorporating these practices into our daily lives, we can cultivate a sense of inner peace, reduce stress and anxiety, and nurture our overall mental health. Start your journey today and discover the healing power of meditation and mindfulness for yourself.

Chapter 3: Yoga for Specific Mental Health Conditions

Yoga for Depression: Finding Inner Balance

In today's fast-paced and demanding world, it is not uncommon for many individuals to struggle with mental health issues such as depression. The constant stress, pressure, and overwhelming responsibilities can take a toll on our emotional well-being. However, there is a powerful tool that can help us find inner balance and alleviate the symptoms of depression – yoga.

Yoga, an ancient practice originating in India, goes beyond physical exercise. It is a holistic approach that integrates the mind, body, and spirit. Through a combination of postures, breathing techniques, and meditation, yoga offers a path towards mental and emotional healing.

Depression is often characterized by feelings of sadness, low energy, and a lack of motivation. Yoga can help combat these symptoms by increasing the production of endorphins, also known as the "feel-good" hormones. Regular yoga practice stimulates the release of these hormones, which can elevate our mood and create a sense of well-being.

One of the key components of yoga for depression is the focus on deep, conscious breathing. Deep breathing exercises, such as pranayama, increase the oxygen supply to our brain and activate the parasympathetic nervous system, which helps induce a state of relaxation. This can reduce anxiety and stress, two common factors that contribute to depression.

In addition to the physical benefits, yoga provides a space for self-reflection and self-acceptance. During yoga practice, we are encouraged to be present in the moment, to observe our thoughts and emotions without judgment. This mindfulness practice can help us develop a more positive outlook, build resilience, and cultivate self-compassion – all essential elements in overcoming depression.

Yoga also offers a supportive community and a sense of belonging. Attending yoga classes or joining yoga groups can provide a safe space to connect with others who may be going through similar struggles. Sharing experiences and finding support from like-minded individuals can be incredibly empowering and can help reduce feelings of isolation and loneliness.

It is important to note that yoga alone may not be a substitute for professional help when it comes to treating depression. However, it can be a powerful complementary tool to support mental health. If you are experiencing depression, it is recommended to consult with a healthcare professional and consider integrating yoga as part of your overall treatment plan.

In conclusion, yoga has the potential to be a transformative practice for individuals struggling with depression. By incorporating yoga into our lives, we can find inner balance, cultivate self-compassion, and nurture our mental health. Whether you are a beginner or an experienced practitioner, yoga offers a path towards healing and a brighter outlook on life. Embrace the power of yoga and embark on a journey of self-discovery, finding solace, and inner peace.

Yoga for Anxiety: Cultivating Calmness

In today's fast-paced and stressful world, anxiety has become a common issue affecting people from all walks of life. From the demands of work to personal relationships and financial pressures, it is no wonder that anxiety has become a prevalent mental health concern. However, there is hope. Yoga, an ancient practice that combines physical postures, breathing techniques, and meditation, has been proven to be an effective tool in managing anxiety and cultivating calmness.

Yoga is not just a physical exercise; it is a holistic approach to healing and well-being. Through the practice of yoga, individuals can tap into their inner resources to find peace and tranquility, even in the midst of chaos. By focusing on the present moment and connecting with the breath, yoga helps to calm the mind and release tension from the body.

One of the main benefits of yoga for anxiety is its ability to activate the relaxation response. When we experience anxiety, our bodies go into fight-or-flight mode, releasing stress hormones that can wreak havoc on our mental and physical health. Yoga counteracts this response by activating the parasympathetic nervous system, which promotes relaxation and reduces stress.

There are specific yoga postures, or asanas, that are particularly beneficial for anxiety. These postures stretch and strengthen the body, releasing tension and helping to quiet the mind. Some recommended asanas for anxiety include child's pose, forward fold, and legs-up-the-wall pose. These poses can be modified to suit individual needs and abilities, making yoga accessible to everyone.

In addition to physical postures, breathing exercises, or pranayama, are an essential aspect of yoga for anxiety. Deep and mindful breathing techniques, such as alternate nostril breathing and belly breathing, can help calm the nervous system and reduce anxiety levels. By focusing on the breath, we can bring ourselves into the present moment and let go of racing thoughts and worries.

Finally, meditation and mindfulness practices are integral components of yoga for anxiety. By cultivating a non-judgmental awareness of the present moment, we can become more attuned to our thoughts and emotions, allowing us to respond to them in a more balanced and compassionate way. Regular meditation practice can help train the mind to let go of anxious thoughts and worries, promoting a greater sense of calmness and tranquility.

In conclusion, yoga is a powerful tool for managing anxiety and nurturing mental health. By incorporating physical postures, breathing exercises, and meditation into our daily lives, we can cultivate a sense of calmness and peace that transcends the challenges of everyday life. Whether you are a seasoned yogi or a beginner, the healing power of yoga is accessible to all. So, roll out your mat, take a deep breath, and embark on a journey of self-discovery and inner peace through the practice of yoga.

Yoga for PTSD: Healing Trauma through Body-Mind Connection

In the modern world, where stress and trauma have become an unfortunate part of many people's lives, it is crucial to explore alternative approaches to healing. One such approach is the powerful practice of yoga, which not only nurtures physical health but also plays a transformative role in mental well-being. In this subchapter, we delve into the profound benefits of yoga for individuals suffering from post-traumatic stress disorder (PTSD), emphasizing the healing potential of the body-mind connection.

PTSD is a complex mental health condition that occurs after experiencing or witnessing a traumatic event. It can manifest as debilitating symptoms such as intrusive thoughts, flashbacks, anxiety, and hypervigilance. Traditional treatments focus primarily on talk therapy and medication. However, yoga offers a holistic approach that integrates the body and mind to facilitate healing.

Yoga is a practice that combines physical postures (asanas), breath control (pranayama), meditation, and mindfulness techniques. By engaging in these practices, individuals with PTSD can create a safe space within themselves to process their trauma, release emotional tension, and cultivate resilience.

The body-mind connection is a fundamental aspect of yoga. Trauma is stored not only in the mind but also in the body, leading to physical and emotional imbalances. Through yoga, individuals learn to reconnect with their bodies, allowing them to release stored trauma and regain a sense of control over their experiences.

Certain yoga poses, such as Child's Pose and Savasana, promote relaxation and help individuals feel grounded. These poses activate the parasympathetic nervous system, counteracting the hyperarousal often experienced by those with PTSD. Simultaneously, pranayama techniques like deep belly breathing can regulate the breath, calming the mind and reducing anxiety.

Mindfulness and meditation practices in yoga are especially beneficial for individuals with PTSD. By cultivating present-moment awareness, individuals can detach from distressing memories or intrusive thoughts, promoting a sense of peace and acceptance. These practices also enhance self-compassion and self-awareness, allowing individuals to develop a healthier relationship with themselves and their trauma.

It is important to note that yoga is not a substitute for traditional therapy but rather a complementary approach that can enhance overall well-being. By incorporating yoga into their healing journey, individuals with PTSD can experience a profound shift in their physical, mental, and emotional states.

Whether you are someone affected by PTSD or a yoga enthusiast seeking a deeper understanding of its benefits, this subchapter aims to provide valuable insights and practical tools for healing. Discover the transformative power of yoga and unlock the potential for healing trauma through the body-mind connection.

Yoga for Addiction Recovery: Rebuilding a Healthy Relationship with Yourself

In today's fast-paced and stressful world, addiction has become an all too common problem that affects people from all walks of life. Whether it's substance abuse, gambling, or even technology addiction, the consequences can be devastating for both the individual and their loved ones. But there is a powerful tool that can aid in the recovery process and help individuals rebuild a healthy relationship with themselves - yoga.

Yoga is not just a physical exercise; it is a holistic practice that combines physical postures, breathing techniques, meditation, and mindfulness. It is a way to reconnect with our bodies, calm our minds, and find inner peace. The benefits of yoga for addiction recovery are numerous and profound, making it an ideal practice to support individuals on their journey towards healing and self-discovery.

One of the key aspects of addiction recovery is rebuilding a healthy relationship with oneself. Addiction often leads to self-destructive behaviors, low self-esteem, and a loss of self-worth. Yoga can help individuals reconnect with their bodies, fostering self-acceptance and self-love. Through the practice of yoga, individuals learn to listen to their bodies, cultivate compassion for themselves, and let go of self-judgment.

The physical postures, or asanas, in yoga help individuals regain strength, flexibility, and balance, both physically and mentally. These postures also release tension and stress stored in the body, providing a sense of relaxation and calm. By practicing yoga regularly, individuals can develop a greater sense of self-awareness and learn to identify and cope with triggers and cravings.

Breathing exercises, or pranayama, are an integral part of yoga and can be particularly beneficial for addiction recovery. Deep, conscious breathing can help individuals regulate their emotions, reduce anxiety and depression, and increase feelings of relaxation and well-being. By focusing on the breath, individuals can learn to control their impulses and make healthier choices.

Meditation and mindfulness practices in yoga teach individuals to stay present in the moment, observe their thoughts and emotions without judgment, and cultivate a sense of inner peace. These practices help individuals develop greater self-awareness, manage stress, and reduce the risk of relapse.

In conclusion, yoga is a powerful tool for addiction recovery, helping individuals rebuild a healthy relationship with themselves. By incorporating yoga into their recovery journey, individuals can cultivate self-acceptance, self-love, and self-awareness. Yoga provides a safe and supportive space for individuals to heal, grow, and find inner peace. So, whether you are struggling with addiction or simply seeking a healthier relationship with yourself, consider incorporating yoga into your life and experience the transformative power it can have on your mental health and overall well-being.

Chapter 4: Yoga for Emotional Healing

Cultivating Self-Compassion through Yoga

Yoga has long been recognized as a transformative practice that not only benefits the physical body but also nurtures the mind and soul. In recent years, there has been a growing interest in the field of mental health and the role that yoga can play in promoting emotional well-being. One aspect of mental health that yoga can greatly impact is self-compassion.

Self-compassion is the practice of treating oneself with kindness, understanding, and acceptance, especially in times of difficulty or failure. It involves acknowledging our own suffering and extending compassion to ourselves, just as we would to a dear friend or loved one. Cultivating self-compassion through yoga can be a powerful tool in nurturing mental health and creating a positive relationship with ourselves.

Yoga teaches us to be present in the moment, to observe our thoughts and feelings without judgment. This mindfulness practice allows us to become aware of our internal dialogue and the way we talk to ourselves. Through yoga, we can start noticing any negative self-talk or self-criticism and gently replace it with compassionate and supportive thoughts.

The physical postures of yoga, known as asanas, also play a significant role in developing self-compassion. Each pose challenges our bodies in different ways, and it is essential to listen to our bodies and honor our limitations. By practicing self-compassion on the mat, we learn to respect our bodies' boundaries, avoid pushing ourselves too hard, and celebrate our progress, no matter how small.

Breathing techniques, or pranayama, are another fundamental aspect of yoga that can aid in cultivating self-compassion. Focusing on deep, slow breaths helps us connect with our bodies, calm our minds, and foster a sense of self-care. By intentionally directing our breath towards areas of tension or discomfort, we can soothe ourselves and offer self-compassion during challenging moments.

Furthermore, yoga philosophy guides us to embrace non-judgment and acceptance, both on and off the mat. Through the practice of yoga, we learn to let go of comparing ourselves to others, to release expectations, and to accept ourselves as we are. This self-acceptance and non-judgment pave the way for self-compassion to flourish.

In conclusion, yoga offers a unique path to cultivating self-compassion. By integrating mindfulness, asanas, pranayama, and yoga philosophy into our practice, we can develop a nurturing relationship with ourselves. The healing power of yoga extends beyond the physical, benefiting our mental health and allowing us to approach life with greater self-compassion. Whether you are a seasoned yogi or just beginning your journey, exploring self-compassion through yoga can be a transformative experience that enhances your overall well-being.

Yoga for Grief and Loss: Nurturing the Healing Process

Grief and loss are universal experiences that touch every one of us at some point in our lives. Whether it is the loss of a loved one, the end of a relationship, the loss of a job, or any other form of loss, the pain can be overwhelming, leaving us feeling lost and broken.

In these moments of deep sorrow, yoga can provide solace and support in nurturing the healing process. The ancient practice of yoga offers a unique and profound way to navigate through the intricate layers of grief. It allows us to find balance, acceptance, and inner peace amidst the rollercoaster of emotions.

Yoga encourages us to connect with our bodies, breath, and minds, enabling us to process and release the intense emotions that accompany grief. Through gentle, flowing movements, we can release physical tension and create space for healing. The practice of asanas (yoga postures) promotes strength, flexibility, and resilience, both physically and emotionally.

Breathing techniques, or pranayama, are an integral part of yoga for grief and loss. Deep, mindful breathing helps calm the nervous system, reduce anxiety, and bring us into the present moment. It allows us to connect with the rhythm of our breath, which can provide a sense of grounding and stability during times of immense pain.

Meditation and mindfulness practices help us cultivate self-awareness and acceptance. By turning inward and observing our thoughts and emotions without judgment, we can begin to unravel the layers of grief. Through meditation, we learn to be present with our pain and develop compassion for ourselves and others who may be experiencing similar struggles.

Yoga also offers a sense of community and support. Joining a yoga class or a grief-specific yoga group allows us to connect with others who are on a similar journey. Sharing our stories, tears, and laughter within a safe space can be immensely healing and provide a sense of belonging.

In the book "The Healing Power of Yoga: Nurturing Mental Health for All," we explore the profound benefits of yoga for grief and loss. We delve into various yoga practices, including asanas, pranayama, meditation, and mindfulness, providing practical guidance and gentle encouragement.

Whether you are new to yoga or have an established practice, this subchapter aims to provide you with tools and techniques to nurture your healing process. It is a gentle reminder that even in the darkest moments of grief, there is light and hope, and yoga can be a powerful and transformative tool on your journey towards healing and wholeness.

Remember, grief is a deeply personal and unique experience, and there is no right or wrong way to navigate it. Yoga offers a compassionate and gentle path towards embracing your grief, honoring your loss, and finding the strength to move forward with love and resilience.

Yoga for Anger Management: Channeling Emotions Positively

In today's fast-paced and demanding world, it's common for individuals to experience feelings of anger and frustration. While anger is a natural emotion, it can become destructive if not managed properly. This subchapter explores the transformative power of yoga as a tool for anger management, offering practical techniques to channel emotions positively and restore inner peace.

Yoga, an ancient practice originating in India, offers a holistic approach to mental and physical well-being. By combining physical postures, breath control, and meditation, yoga cultivates self-awareness, mindfulness, and emotional balance. It provides a safe and non-judgmental space to explore and understand our emotions, including anger.

Anger often arises from unmet expectations, stress, or unresolved conflicts. Through yoga, one can develop a deeper understanding of the underlying causes of anger and learn to respond rather than react to challenging situations. By engaging in regular yoga practice, individuals can build resilience and cultivate a greater sense of calmness, compassion, and empathy.

Physical postures, or asanas, play a vital role in anger management. Certain poses, such as the Warrior series, help release tension and promote a sense of strength and empowerment. Twisting poses, like the seated spinal twist, aid in detoxifying the body and releasing stagnant energy. These postures not only release physical tension but also help release emotional blockages, allowing individuals to let go of anger and negativity.

Breath control, known as pranayama, is another powerful tool in anger management. By consciously regulating the breath, individuals can soothe the nervous system and create a sense of calmness. Deep abdominal breathing and alternate nostril breathing are particularly effective in reducing anger and promoting emotional balance.

Meditation, the cornerstone of yoga, allows individuals to observe and detach from their anger. By cultivating a state of stillness and inner silence, one can gain clarity and perspective on their emotions. Meditation techniques, such as loving-kindness meditation or mindfulness meditation, enable individuals to develop self-compassion, forgiveness, and acceptance.

In conclusion, yoga offers a holistic approach to anger management, empowering individuals to channel their emotions positively. By integrating physical postures, breath control, and meditation into their daily lives, individuals can cultivate self-awareness, resilience, and emotional balance. Whether you are a seasoned yogi or a beginner, the healing power of yoga is accessible to everyone, offering a path towards nurturing mental health and well-being.

Yoga for Enhancing Emotional Resilience

In today's fast-paced and stress-filled world, it's crucial to prioritize our mental health and emotional well-being. Yoga, an ancient practice originating from India, offers a holistic approach to nurturing our mental health and building emotional resilience. Whether you're a yoga enthusiast or new to the practice, incorporating yoga into your daily routine can greatly benefit your emotional well-being.

Emotional resilience refers to our ability to adapt and bounce back from challenges, setbacks, and stressors. It's about cultivating inner strength and a positive mindset to navigate life's ups and downs. Yoga provides us with a powerful toolkit to enhance our emotional resilience and promote a sense of calm, balance, and stability.

One of the key ways yoga enhances emotional resilience is through the connection between mind, body, and breath. The practice of yoga asanas (postures) promotes physical strength, flexibility, and balance. As we move through the poses, we cultivate mindfulness and focus on our breath, allowing us to tune into our body's sensations and become more aware of our emotions. This increased awareness helps us recognize and process our feelings more effectively.

Additionally, yoga incorporates mindfulness and meditation practices, which are known to reduce stress and anxiety. By practicing mindfulness, we learn to observe our thoughts and emotions without judgment, creating space for self-reflection and self-compassion. This ability to stay present in the moment and accept our emotions empowers us to better manage stressful situations and build emotional resilience.

Furthermore, yoga encourages the release of emotional tension and promotes relaxation. Through deep breathing exercises and gentle stretching, we activate the body's relaxation response, calming the nervous system and reducing the impact of stress on our emotional well-being. Regular yoga practice can improve sleep quality, boost mood, and decrease symptoms of depression and anxiety.

Yoga is for everyone, regardless of age, fitness level, or previous experience. Whether you prefer a vigorous vinyasa flow or a gentle restorative practice, there are numerous yoga styles and classes available to suit your needs. It's essential to find a qualified yoga instructor who can guide you safely and provide modifications as needed.

Incorporating yoga into your daily routine can significantly enhance your emotional resilience. The Healing Power of Yoga: Nurturing Mental Health for All encourages readers to explore the practice of yoga and witness the transformative effects it can have on their emotional well-being. Start your journey towards emotional resilience today by stepping onto the mat and embracing the healing power of yoga.

Chapter 5: Incorporating Yoga into Daily Life for Mental Wellbeing

Yoga for Better Sleep: Promoting Restful Nights

In today's fast-paced and hectic world, getting a good night's sleep is more important than ever. Lack of sleep can lead to a range of health issues, including increased stress levels, decreased productivity, and even mental health disorders. Fortunately, yoga offers a natural and effective solution to promote restful nights and improve the quality of sleep for everyone.

Yoga, an ancient practice that combines physical postures, breathing techniques, and meditation, has been scientifically proven to reduce stress and anxiety, calm the mind, and relax the body. By incorporating specific yoga poses and practices into your daily routine, you can create a bedtime ritual that will help you unwind, release tension, and prepare your body and mind for a peaceful sleep.

One of the most effective yoga practices for better sleep is a gentle and slow-paced sequence of postures known as restorative yoga. This style of yoga focuses on deep relaxation and rejuvenation, allowing you to let go of physical and mental tension. Restorative poses, such as supported child's pose, legs up the wall, and reclining bound angle pose, promote relaxation by gently stretching and opening the body, while also slowing down the breath and calming the mind.

In addition to specific yoga poses, breathing exercises, or pranayama, can also play a crucial role in promoting better sleep. Techniques like alternate nostril breathing and deep belly breathing activate the body's relaxation response, helping to reduce stress and induce a state of calmness before bed.

Furthermore, incorporating mindfulness meditation into your bedtime routine can be highly beneficial for promoting restful nights. Mindfulness meditation involves bringing your attention to the present moment, observing your thoughts and sensations without judgment. By practicing mindfulness, you can quiet the mind, let go of worries, and cultivate a sense of inner peace, all of which contribute to a more restful sleep.

Remember, yoga is a personal journey, and it's essential to listen to your body and find the practices that work best for you. By embracing yoga as a tool for better sleep, you can create a bedtime routine that nurtures your mental health and promotes restful nights for all. So, roll out your yoga mat, take a deep breath, and embark on a journey towards a more peaceful and rejuvenating sleep.

Yoga for Work-Life Balance: Finding Harmony amidst Chaos

In today's fast-paced and demanding world, achieving work-life balance seems like an elusive dream. The constant juggling between professional responsibilities and personal obligations often takes a toll on our mental and physical well-being. However, the ancient practice of yoga holds the key to finding harmony amidst the chaos and nurturing our mental health.

Yoga is not just a physical exercise; it is a holistic approach to life that encompasses physical postures (asanas), breathing techniques (pranayama), and meditation. Through the regular practice of yoga, we can cultivate a sense of calmness, clarity, and balance that transcends into all aspects of our lives.

One of the greatest benefits of yoga is its ability to alleviate stress and anxiety. By engaging in mindful movements and deep breathing, we activate the parasympathetic nervous system, which counteracts the fight-or-flight response. This helps us relax, release tension, and restore our energy levels. Yoga also enhances our ability to focus and concentrate, enabling us to be more productive and efficient in our professional lives.

Moreover, yoga teaches us the art of surrendering and letting go. In a world where we are constantly striving and pushing ourselves to achieve more, yoga reminds us to embrace stillness and find contentment in the present moment. By cultivating this mindset, we can detach ourselves from the pressures of work and allow ourselves to fully enjoy our personal lives.

Finding work-life balance through yoga also involves setting boundaries and prioritizing self-care. Yoga encourages us to listen to our bodies and honor our limitations. By incorporating regular yoga practice into our daily routines, we create a space for self-reflection, self-care, and self-compassion. This, in turn, allows us to show up as our best selves in both our personal and professional relationships.

Whether you are a busy professional, a parent juggling multiple responsibilities, or someone seeking inner peace, yoga can benefit everyone. It is a versatile practice that can be tailored to individual needs and schedules. Even a few minutes of yoga each day can make a significant difference in restoring balance and promoting mental well-being.

In conclusion, yoga offers a powerful tool for finding work-life balance and nurturing our mental health. By incorporating yoga into our lives, we can navigate the chaos with grace and cultivate inner harmony. So, take a deep breath, roll out your yoga mat, and embark on a journey of self-discovery and healing. The rewards are boundless, and the path to work-life balance awaits you.

Yoga for Improved Concentration and Focus

In today's fast-paced and demanding world, it is increasingly challenging to stay mentally focused and maintain a high level of concentration. Our minds are constantly bombarded with distractions, making it difficult to complete tasks and achieve our goals effectively. However, by incorporating yoga into our daily routine, we can cultivate improved concentration and focus, allowing us to navigate through life with a clear and centered mind.

Yoga, an ancient practice that harmonizes the mind, body, and spirit, offers a multitude of techniques that can enhance our ability to concentrate and focus. Through the gentle movements, controlled breathing, and meditation, yoga helps us develop a heightened sense of self-awareness, enabling us to better control our thoughts and emotions.

One of the primary ways yoga improves concentration is through the use of asanas, or yoga postures. Asanas require us to focus on our breath and bodily sensations, grounding us in the present moment. By holding poses and maintaining balance, we learn to quiet the mind and tune out distractions, fostering a deep sense of concentration.

Pranayama, the practice of controlled breathing, is another powerful tool within the realm of yoga. Deep, slow breathing techniques, such as the alternate nostril breathing or the three-part breath, help calm the mind, reduce stress, and increase oxygen flow to the brain. This enhanced oxygenation promotes mental clarity, sharpness, and improved focus.

Furthermore, meditation plays a vital role in enhancing concentration and focus. By training the mind to remain in the present moment, meditation allows us to let go of racing thoughts and worries. Through regular practice, we gain the ability to observe our thoughts without judgment, creating mental space and improving our ability to concentrate on the task at hand.

Incorporating yoga into our daily routine can significantly benefit individuals of all ages and backgrounds. Whether you are a student struggling to concentrate on your studies, a professional aiming to increase productivity, or someone simply seeking mental clarity and focus, yoga can offer immense support.

By making yoga a regular practice, you will gradually experience improved concentration, heightened productivity, and a greater sense of mental well-being. Embrace the healing power of yoga and witness the transformative effects it can have on your ability to maintain focus and achieve mental clarity in all aspects of your life.

Yoga for Self-Care: Nurturing Your Mental Health

In today's fast-paced and stressful world, taking care of our mental health has become more important than ever. With the constant demands and pressures of daily life, it's easy to neglect our emotional well-being. However, incorporating yoga into your self-care routine can be a powerful tool for nurturing your mental health.

Yoga, an ancient practice that originated in India, is not just a physical exercise. It is a holistic approach that combines breath control, meditation, and asanas (poses) to create a sense of balance and harmony within the mind, body, and spirit. By incorporating yoga into your self-care routine, you can experience numerous mental health benefits.

One of the key benefits of yoga for mental health is stress reduction. The practice of yoga helps activate the parasympathetic nervous system, which promotes relaxation and reduces the production of stress hormones. Through deep breathing techniques and gentle movements, yoga encourages you to be present in the moment and let go of worries and anxieties.

Moreover, yoga can improve your overall mood and emotional well-being. Regular yoga practice increases the production of serotonin, a neurotransmitter known as the "feel-good" hormone. This can help alleviate symptoms of depression and anxiety, promoting a more positive outlook on life.

Yoga also provides a safe space for self-reflection and self-acceptance. By turning inward and focusing on your breath and body, you can cultivate mindfulness and self-awareness. This allows you to observe your thoughts and emotions without judgment, fostering a sense of compassion and understanding towards yourself.

Additionally, yoga can enhance your resilience and ability to cope with life's challenges. Through challenging poses and balancing exercises, you learn to stay steady and calm in difficult situations. This can translate into your everyday life, helping you navigate stressors with grace and equanimity.

Incorporating yoga into your self-care routine doesn't require a significant time commitment. Even just a few minutes of gentle stretching and deep breathing can make a difference in your mental well-being. Whether you choose to practice at home or join a yoga class, make self-care through yoga a priority and witness the transformative power it can have on your mental health.

Remember, self-care is essential for everyone, regardless of age, gender, or fitness level. Embrace the healing power of yoga and give yourself the gift of nurturing your mental health.

Chapter 6: The Science behind Yoga and Mental Health

The Neurological Benefits of Yoga

Yoga is often revered for its physical benefits, such as increased flexibility and strength, but its positive impact on mental health is equally remarkable. In recent years, scientific research has shed light on the neurological benefits of practicing yoga, making it an increasingly popular tool for promoting overall well-being.

One of the key neurological benefits of yoga is its ability to reduce stress and anxiety. In today's fast-paced world, stress has become a common and debilitating issue for many individuals. Yoga, with its focus on deep breathing and mindfulness, activates the body's relaxation response and helps to calm the mind. This triggers a decrease in the production of stress hormones, such as cortisol, and promotes the release of feel-good neurotransmitters like serotonin and dopamine. As a result, practitioners often experience reduced anxiety levels and an improved sense of well-being.

Furthermore, regular yoga practice has been shown to enhance cognitive function and memory. Studies have found that yoga increases the volume of the hippocampus - a part of the brain crucial for memory formation and retention. Additionally, yoga stimulates the prefrontal cortex, which is responsible for executive functions like decision-making, attention, and problem-solving. By engaging in yoga regularly, individuals can enhance their cognitive abilities and improve their overall mental clarity.

In addition to reducing stress and enhancing cognitive function, yoga has been found to be an effective tool for managing and even preventing neurological disorders. Research suggests that yoga can help individuals with conditions such as Parkinson's disease, multiple sclerosis, and epilepsy by improving balance, coordination, and motor function. The mind-body connection established through yoga practice is believed to play a significant role in these improvements.

For individuals struggling with depression, yoga can provide a much-needed boost to their mental health. Yoga's emphasis on deep breathing and gentle movements helps to increase the production of gamma-aminobutyric acid (GABA), a neurotransmitter that promotes feelings of relaxation and happiness. This can alleviate symptoms of depression and contribute to a more positive outlook on life.

In conclusion, the neurological benefits of yoga are undeniable. By reducing stress, enhancing cognitive function, and aiding in the management of neurological disorders, yoga has the power to nurture mental health for individuals from all walks of life. Whether you are a seasoned yogi or a beginner, incorporating yoga into your routine can make a significant difference in your overall well-being. So unroll your mat, take a deep breath, and embark on a journey towards a healthier mind and body through the transformative power of yoga.

Understanding the Role of Yoga in Stress Reduction

In today's fast-paced and demanding world, stress has become an inevitable part of our lives. From work pressures to personal challenges, stress can take a toll on our mental health and overall well-being. Fortunately, there is a powerful tool that can help us combat stress and find balance in our lives - yoga.

Yoga, an ancient practice originating in India, has gained immense popularity worldwide for its numerous physical and mental health benefits. While many perceive yoga as a physical exercise, its true essence lies in its ability to bring about a deep sense of peace and relaxation. In fact, one of yoga's primary objectives is to calm the mind and reduce stress.

So, how does yoga help in stress reduction? Firstly, yoga incorporates various breathing techniques, known as pranayama, which have a direct impact on our nervous system. Deep and mindful breathing activates the parasympathetic nervous system, triggering the relaxation response and reducing the production of stress hormones such as cortisol. By practicing pranayama regularly, individuals can train their bodies to respond more calmly to stressful situations.

Furthermore, yoga involves a series of physical postures, known as asanas, that not only enhance flexibility and strength but also promote relaxation. These asanas are designed to release tension from the body, allowing for the free flow of energy and reducing physical manifestations of stress, such as headaches and muscle tension. Additionally, the practice of asanas requires a heightened sense of awareness, diverting the mind's focus from stressful thoughts and promoting a state of mindfulness and presence.

In addition to pranayama and asanas, meditation plays a crucial role in stress reduction through yoga. Meditation is a practice of training the mind to focus and redirect thoughts. By practicing meditation regularly, individuals can cultivate a calm and clear mind, enabling them to better cope with stressors and maintain mental well-being.

Yoga is not only a powerful stress reduction tool but also a holistic approach to overall health and well-being. Regular practice of yoga can improve sleep quality, boost immunity, and enhance emotional resilience. It is accessible to people of all ages and fitness levels, making it a versatile practice suitable for everyone.

In conclusion, understanding the role of yoga in stress reduction is essential in today's fast-paced world. By incorporating yoga into our lives, we can harness its healing power to nurture our mental health and find inner peace. Whether you are new to yoga or a seasoned practitioner, embracing this ancient practice can help you navigate through life's challenges with greater ease and harmony.

Yoga and the Mind-Body Connection

In today's fast-paced world, it is becoming increasingly important to find ways to restore balance and nurture our mental health. One practice that has gained immense popularity in recent years is yoga. Yoga is not just a physical exercise; it is a holistic approach to well-being that encompasses the mind, body, and spirit. One of the core principles of yoga is the mind-body connection, which emphasizes the interdependence and inseparability of our mental and physical states.

The mind-body connection is a concept that has been recognized by ancient civilizations for centuries. However, it is only in recent years that modern science has started to explore and acknowledge its significance. Research has shown that our mental and emotional states can have a profound impact on our physical health, and vice versa. Yoga, with its focus on mindfulness and breath awareness, provides a powerful tool for enhancing this mind-body connection.

Through the practice of yoga, we learn to cultivate a deep sense of awareness and presence in the present moment. By paying attention to our breath, sensations, and thoughts, we can begin to understand the intricate relationship between our mind and body. As we move through the various yoga poses, or asanas, we become more attuned to the sensations and energy flowing through our bodies. This heightened awareness allows us to identify areas of tension or discomfort and work towards releasing them.

Yoga also encourages us to observe and manage our thoughts and emotions. By practicing mindfulness and meditation, we can develop a greater understanding of our mental patterns and learn to respond to challenges with clarity and calmness. This ability to regulate our emotions and thoughts can have a significant impact on our overall well-being, as it helps us to reduce stress, anxiety, and depression.

The mind-body connection in yoga goes beyond the mat. The principles and practices we learn on the yoga mat can be applied to our daily lives, enabling us to navigate challenges with resilience and grace. By fostering a strong mind-body connection, we can enhance our physical health, improve our mental well-being, and cultivate a greater sense of inner peace and harmony.

Whether you are a seasoned yogi or new to the practice, exploring the mind-body connection in yoga can be a transformative journey. By embracing this holistic approach to well-being, you can unlock the healing power of yoga and nurture your mental health for all. So, take a deep breath, step onto your mat, and embark on this incredible journey of self-discovery and transformation. Your mind and body will thank you for it.

Exploring the Psychological Effects of Yoga

Yoga is often associated with physical fitness and flexibility, but its benefits extend far beyond the physical realm. In recent years, researchers and mental health professionals have started to recognize and explore the profound psychological effects of practicing yoga. From reducing stress and anxiety to improving mood and overall mental well-being, yoga has emerged as a powerful tool for nurturing mental health.

One of the most well-known psychological benefits of yoga is its ability to reduce stress. In today's fast-paced world, stress has become a common occurrence, leading to various mental health issues. However, through a combination of physical postures, breath control, and meditation, yoga helps activate the body's relaxation response, promoting a state of calmness and reducing stress levels. Regular practice of yoga has been shown to lower cortisol levels, the hormone associated with stress, thereby improving overall mental well-being.

Furthermore, yoga has been found to alleviate symptoms of anxiety and depression. By focusing on breath control and mindfulness, yoga encourages individuals to stay present in the moment, diverting their attention from negative thoughts and worries. This mindfulness aspect of yoga helps individuals develop a better understanding of their emotions and thoughts, leading to increased self-awareness and emotional regulation. Studies have shown that yoga can be as effective as traditional forms of therapy in reducing symptoms of anxiety and depression.

In addition to stress reduction and mood improvement, yoga also enhances cognitive functioning. Regular yoga practice has been found to improve memory, attention, and concentration. This is attributed to the combination of physical movement, breathwork, and meditation, which increase blood flow to the brain and promote neural connectivity. These cognitive benefits make yoga a valuable practice for individuals of all ages, from students looking to improve their academic performance to older adults aiming to maintain mental sharpness.

Moreover, practicing yoga in a group setting fosters a sense of community and social connection. This can be especially beneficial for individuals struggling with feelings of loneliness or isolation. The supportive environment of a yoga class promotes social interaction and provides a sense of belonging, which in turn positively impacts mental health.

In conclusion, the psychological effects of yoga are vast and transformative. From reducing stress and anxiety to improving mood and cognitive functioning, yoga offers a holistic approach to nurturing mental health. Whether you are a seasoned yogi or a beginner, incorporating yoga into your daily routine can bring about positive psychological changes that benefit everyone, regardless of age or background. Embrace the healing power of yoga and embark on a journey of self-discovery and mental well-being.

Chapter 7: Creating a Personalized Yoga Practice for Mental Health

Setting Intentions and Goals for Your Yoga Journey

Embarking on a yoga journey is not just about the physical practice; it is a holistic experience that nurtures our mental health and overall well-being. As you step onto your mat, it is important to set intentions and goals to guide you on this transformative path. Whether you are a beginner or an experienced yogi, this subchapter will help you understand the importance of setting intentions and goals in your yoga practice.

Setting intentions is a way to bring conscious awareness to your practice. It helps you align your mind, body, and spirit, creating a deeper connection with yourself and the present moment. By setting intentions, you are essentially planting seeds of positivity and purpose in your practice. It could be as simple as cultivating gratitude, finding inner peace, or letting go of stress and negativity. Your intentions will shape the energy and focus of your practice, allowing you to dive deeper into the essence of yoga.

Goals, on the other hand, provide a roadmap for your yoga journey. They give you something to strive for and help you measure your progress along the way. Whether you aim to master a challenging pose, increase flexibility, or find balance in your life, goals provide direction and motivation. It is important to set realistic and achievable goals that align with your current abilities and aspirations. Remember that yoga is a personal journey, and your goals should reflect your unique needs and desires.

When setting intentions and goals, it is crucial to approach them with compassion and self-acceptance. Yoga is not about competition or comparison; it is about embracing your own journey and honoring where you are in the present moment. Be gentle with yourself and allow room for growth and transformation. Celebrate even the smallest accomplishments and milestones along the way.

As you embark on your yoga journey, take the time to reflect on your intentions and set meaningful goals. Write them down and revisit them regularly to stay focused and motivated. Allow your intentions and goals to guide you on and off the mat, bringing balance, peace, and well-being into your life.

Remember, your yoga journey is unique to you. Embrace the process, trust in yourself, and let the healing power of yoga nurture your mental health and well-being. Namaste.

Designing a Yoga Routine for Mental Wellbeing

Yoga is not just a physical practice; it is a holistic approach that nurtures the mind, body, and soul. In today's fast-paced and stressful world, maintaining mental wellbeing is crucial for everyone. Incorporating yoga into your daily routine can be a powerful tool to cultivate mental resilience, find inner peace, and promote overall mental health.

Creating a yoga routine tailored to support mental wellbeing does not require any prior experience or expertise. It simply requires an open mind, willingness to explore, and commitment to self-care. Here are some key considerations to keep in mind when designing a yoga routine for mental wellbeing.

1. Set an Intention: Begin by setting an intention for your yoga practice. Reflect on what you hope to achieve mentally or emotionally through your practice. Whether it's finding calm, reducing anxiety, or improving focus, setting an intention will guide your practice and keep you aligned with your goals.

2. Breathwork: Incorporate breathwork or pranayama techniques into your routine. Breath is a powerful tool to regulate the nervous system and calm the mind. Explore techniques such as deep belly breathing, alternate nostril breathing, or the 4-7-8 breath to cultivate a sense of mental tranquility.

3. Mindfulness and Meditation: Dedicate a portion of your practice to mindfulness and meditation. These practices enhance self-awareness, reduce stress, and promote emotional balance. Experiment with

guided meditations, body scans, or simply sitting in stillness and observing your thoughts without judgment.

4. Gentle Asanas: Choose gentle yoga asanas (poses) that focus on stretching, relaxation, and grounding. Incorporate poses such as child's pose, seated forward fold, gentle twists, and legs-up-the-wall pose. These poses help release tension, calm the nervous system, and cultivate a sense of wellbeing.

5. Yoga Nidra: Consider including Yoga Nidra, also known as yogic sleep, in your routine. Yoga Nidra is a guided relaxation technique that promotes deep relaxation and rejuvenation. It helps reduce anxiety, improve sleep quality, and restore mental energy.

6. Gratitude Practice: End your yoga routine with a gratitude practice. Take a few moments to reflect on the things you are grateful for. Cultivating gratitude shifts our focus from negativity to positivity, promoting mental wellbeing and contentment.

Remember, there is no right or wrong way to design a yoga routine for mental wellbeing. It is a personal journey of self-discovery and self-care. Listen to your body, honor your limitations, and adapt the practice to suit your needs. As you embark on this journey, be patient and compassionate with yourself. With regular practice, you will gradually experience the profound healing power of yoga on your mental wellbeing.

Adapting Yoga Practices to Fit Your Needs and Abilities

Yoga is a transformative practice that has been celebrated for its ability to improve physical strength, flexibility, and mental well-being. However, it is important to remember that yoga is not a one-size-fits-all practice. Each individual is unique, with different needs, abilities, and limitations. Therefore, it is crucial to adapt yoga practices to fit your own specific requirements.

When beginning your yoga journey, it is important to assess your physical abilities and limitations. If you have any pre-existing medical conditions or injuries, it is essential to consult with a healthcare professional before starting any new exercise regimen. They can provide valuable guidance and help you determine which yoga poses and practices are suitable for your individual needs.

One of the great things about yoga is its versatility. There are various styles and modifications available, making it accessible to people of all fitness levels and ages. If you are a beginner or have limited flexibility, starting with gentle and beginner-friendly yoga classes can be extremely beneficial. These classes will introduce you to foundational poses and teach you proper alignment and breathing techniques.

As you progress in your practice, you may find that certain poses or sequences are challenging for you. This is where modifications come into play. Yoga instructors are trained to provide modifications for different poses, allowing you to customize your practice based on your abilities. For example, if you are unable to perform a full Chaturanga (low plank) pose, you can modify it by performing the pose on your knees instead.

Additionally, props such as blocks, straps, and blankets can be used to support and enhance your practice. These props can help you maintain proper alignment, increase stability, and provide support during challenging poses. Using props is not a sign of weakness or lack of ability; it is a tool to help you achieve the full benefits of each pose safely and comfortably.

Remember, yoga is a personal journey. It is not a competition, nor is it about comparing yourself to others. Listen to your body and honor its limits. Be patient with yourself and embrace the process of growth and self-discovery. With time and dedication, you will witness the positive effects of yoga on your mental and physical well-being.

In conclusion, adapting yoga practices to fit your needs and abilities is essential for a safe and enjoyable practice. By consulting with professionals, starting with beginner-friendly classes, and utilizing modifications and props, you can create a yoga practice that is tailored to your individual requirements. Embrace the journey, and let the healing power of yoga nurture your mental health and well-being.

Seeking Guidance and Support for Your Yoga Practice

Yoga has become increasingly popular in recent years, with people from all walks of life embracing its physical and mental benefits. Whether you are a seasoned yogi or just starting out on your yoga journey, seeking guidance and support can greatly enhance your practice. In this subchapter, we will explore the various ways you can find the assistance you need to nurture and deepen your yoga practice.

One of the most important aspects of seeking guidance is finding a knowledgeable and experienced yoga teacher. A good teacher can provide you with proper alignment cues, help you modify poses for your body, and offer personalized guidance based on your unique needs and goals. Look for a teacher who creates a welcoming and inclusive atmosphere, where you feel comfortable asking questions and seeking clarification. Remember, yoga is a lifelong practice, and finding the right teacher can make all the difference in your progress and enjoyment.

In addition to finding a skilled teacher, joining a yoga community or studio can offer tremendous support and inspiration. Connecting with like-minded individuals who share your passion for yoga can provide a sense of belonging and encouragement. Engage in conversations, attend workshops, and participate in group classes to broaden your knowledge and deepen your practice. Many studios also offer mentorship programs, where you can receive one-on-one guidance from experienced practitioners, further enhancing your growth.

Beyond the physical practice, seeking guidance for the mental and emotional aspects of yoga is equally important. Yoga is not only about the postures but also about cultivating mindfulness, self-awareness, and inner peace. Consider exploring meditation classes, yoga philosophy workshops, or mindfulness retreats to dive deeper into these aspects of yoga. These practices can help you develop a deeper understanding of yourself and provide tools for managing stress, anxiety, and other mental health challenges.

Finally, do not underestimate the power of self-study and self-reflection in your yoga practice. Journaling, reading books on yoga and spirituality, and exploring online resources can be invaluable in deepening your understanding and expanding your practice. Remember that yoga is a personal journey, and seeking guidance and support can come from within as well.

In conclusion, seeking guidance and support for your yoga practice is essential for growth and transformation. Whether it is through finding a skilled teacher, joining a yoga community, exploring the mental and emotional aspects, or engaging in self-study, nurturing your yoga practice will bring immense benefits to your overall well-being. Embrace the journey, seek guidance, and watch as your practice unfolds and transforms your life.

Chapter 8: Overcoming Challenges and Sustaining a Yoga Practice for Mental Health

Dealing with Resistance and Self-Doubt

In the journey towards nurturing mental health, it is common to encounter resistance and self-doubt. These obstacles can arise when engaging in any practice, including yoga. However, it is important to remember that these challenges are a normal part of the process and can be overcome with patience, perseverance, and self-compassion.

Resistance often manifests as a reluctance to start or continue a yoga practice. It may stem from fear of the unknown, a lack of confidence, or a sense of being overwhelmed by the physical and mental demands of yoga. When faced with resistance, it is crucial to acknowledge and honor the feelings that arise. Take a moment to reflect on the underlying reasons for resistance. Is it a fear of failure? Are there limiting beliefs about one's abilities? By identifying the root cause, it becomes easier to address and overcome resistance.

Self-doubt, on the other hand, can be a constant companion throughout the yoga journey. It is the nagging voice that tells us we are not good enough or capable of achieving our goals. Self-doubt can be paralyzing, preventing us from fully experiencing the transformative power of yoga. To combat self-doubt, it is essential to cultivate self-compassion and adopt a growth mindset. Recognize that everyone starts somewhere, and progress is not linear. Celebrate small victories and focus on personal growth rather than comparing oneself to others. Remember that yoga is a practice, and it is through consistent effort and patience that progress is made.

When faced with resistance and self-doubt, it can be helpful to seek support from the yoga community. Surrounding oneself with like-minded individuals who have experienced similar challenges can provide encouragement and motivation. Consider joining a yoga class, participating in online forums, or connecting with a mentor or teacher who can offer guidance and support.

Ultimately, dealing with resistance and self-doubt is an opportunity for personal growth and transformation. Embrace these challenges as part of the yoga journey, and approach them with kindness and curiosity. By persisting through resistance and cultivating self-belief, one can tap into the healing power of yoga and nurture their mental health. Remember, you are capable, and your journey is unique and worthwhile.

Overcoming Physical Limitations and Modifications in Yoga

Yoga is a holistic practice that benefits the mind, body, and spirit. It has gained immense popularity worldwide, with people from all walks of life embracing its transformative power. However, it is essential to acknowledge that not everyone has the same physical abilities or flexibility levels. This subchapter aims to explore how individuals can overcome physical limitations and make modifications in their yoga practice to suit their unique needs.

Yoga is a practice that is adaptable to all bodies, regardless of age, size, or physical condition. It is crucial to remember that yoga is not about achieving perfect poses but rather about finding balance and harmony within oneself. With this mindset, individuals with physical limitations can embark on their yoga journey with confidence.

One of the first steps in overcoming physical limitations in yoga is to listen to your body. Every individual's body is unique, and it is essential to honor its limitations and boundaries. By paying attention to sensations and any discomfort, modifications can be made to poses to ensure safety and prevent injury. For example, if a person has limited mobility in their knees, they can use props like blocks or bolsters to support their body in a modified version of a pose.

Another way to overcome physical limitations is to work with a knowledgeable and experienced yoga instructor. A qualified instructor can guide individuals in making appropriate modifications and offer alternative poses that cater to their specific needs. They can also provide valuable insights on how to build strength, flexibility, and endurance gradually, allowing individuals to progress at their own pace.

Additionally, it is vital to cultivate a compassionate mindset towards oneself. Comparing one's practice to others or feeling discouraged by physical limitations can hinder progress. Instead, individuals should focus on their own journey and celebrate the small victories along the way. Yoga is a personal practice, and each step forward, no matter how small, is a significant achievement.

In conclusion, yoga is a practice that can be adapted to suit the needs of individuals with physical limitations. By listening to their bodies, working with knowledgeable instructors, and cultivating self-compassion, individuals can overcome physical barriers and experience the healing power of yoga. Remember, yoga is for everyone, and with modifications, it can become a transformative practice that nurtures mental health and overall well-being.

Maintaining Motivation and Consistency in Your Practice

Introduction:

In the fast-paced world we live in, finding the motivation and consistency to maintain a regular yoga practice can be challenging. However, the benefits of yoga on our mental health make it worth the effort. This subchapter aims to provide inspiration and practical tips to help everyone, regardless of their level of experience, stay motivated and consistent in their yoga practice.

1. Understanding the Power of Yoga:

Yoga is not just a physical exercise; it is a holistic practice that nurtures mental health. By combining physical postures, breathing techniques, and meditation, yoga helps us find balance, reduce stress, and cultivate a sense of inner peace. Recognizing the immense benefits that yoga offers to our overall well-being can serve as a powerful motivator to maintain a consistent practice.

2. Setting Realistic Goals:

When starting or restarting a yoga practice, it is important to set realistic goals. Begin with small, achievable targets that fit into your lifestyle. For instance, committing to a 10-minute daily practice in the morning or attending one yoga class per week can be a great starting point. As you experience the positive effects of your practice, you can gradually increase your goals.

3. Creating a Sacred Space:

Designate a specific area in your home as your yoga space. This can be a corner of a room or a separate room entirely. Decorate it with items that promote relaxation and tranquility, such as candles, incense, or soothing music. Having a dedicated space for your practice creates a sense of sacredness and makes it easier to mentally transition into the yoga mindset.

4. Prioritizing Self-Care:

Make self-care a priority by scheduling your yoga practice into your daily routine. Treat it as an essential appointment with yourself, just like you would with any other commitment. By prioritizing your practice, you are acknowledging the importance of your mental health and setting boundaries to ensure consistency.

5. Exploring Various Styles:

To keep your practice fresh and exciting, explore different styles of yoga. From Hatha to Vinyasa, Yin to Ashtanga, there are numerous styles to choose from. Experimenting with different classes or online videos can help you discover what resonates with you the most. Variety prevents monotony and keeps your motivation levels high.

Conclusion:

Maintaining motivation and consistency in your yoga practice requires dedication and perseverance. By understanding the power of yoga, setting realistic goals, creating a sacred space, prioritizing self-care, and exploring different styles, you can overcome the challenges and reap the mental health benefits that yoga offers. Remember, every small step towards consistency is a step towards nurturing your mental well-being.

Building a Supportive Community for Continued Growth

In the journey towards nurturing mental health and well-being, building a supportive community is crucial. This holds true for everyone, regardless of age, background, or level of yoga practice. Yoga, with its holistic approach to health and mindfulness, has the potential to bring people together and create a nurturing environment for continued growth.

When individuals come together to practice yoga, they form a bond that goes beyond the physical postures. The shared experience of exploring the mind-body connection and the accompanying sense of vulnerability can foster a sense of belonging and understanding. This community becomes a safe space where individuals can express themselves, share their struggles, and find support from like-minded individuals.

One of the key factors in building a supportive community is creating an inclusive environment. Yoga should be accessible to everyone, regardless of their physical abilities or previous experience. By offering modifications and variations, yoga teachers can ensure that all participants feel welcome and encouraged. This inclusivity also extends beyond the physical practice, as individuals from diverse backgrounds and cultures come together to learn and grow.

Within this supportive community, individuals can find inspiration and motivation to continue their yoga journey. Seeing others overcome challenges, achieve personal growth, or simply find solace in their practice can be incredibly empowering. Sharing these experiences and celebrating each other's progress fosters a sense of camaraderie and reinforces the belief that everyone is capable of growth and transformation.

In addition to the physical practice, a supportive yoga community also emphasizes the importance of mental health. Creating space for open discussions on topics such as stress management, self-care, and mindfulness techniques can help individuals develop a deeper understanding of their own mental well-being. This encourages a sense of empathy and compassion towards others and provides a platform for sharing resources and strategies for maintaining mental health.

Ultimately, building a supportive community for continued growth in yoga involves creating an environment where individuals feel accepted, inspired, and supported on their journey towards mental well-being. By fostering inclusivity, celebrating each other's progress, and prioritizing mental health, this community becomes a powerful force in nurturing the overall well-being of its members. It is through this collective effort that the healing power of yoga can truly be harnessed for the benefit of all.

Conclusion: Embracing the Healing Power of Yoga for Mental Health

Reflecting on Your Journey and Achievements

In the fast-paced world we live in, it is often challenging to take a moment and reflect on our personal journeys and achievements. However, this self-reflection is a crucial aspect of our overall well-being and personal growth. As we delve deeper into the practice of yoga, it becomes essential to pause and contemplate the transformative power it has had on our mental health and overall life.

Yoga is not just a physical exercise; it is a path towards self-discovery and self-realization. Through the practice of asanas, pranayama, and meditation, we embark on a journey of self-exploration that allows us to connect with our inner selves on a profound level. By dedicating time to reflect on our journey and the achievements we have made along the way, we can gain a deeper understanding of our own progress and the impact yoga has had on our mental health.

When reflecting on your journey, take a moment to acknowledge the challenges you have faced and the milestones you have achieved. Perhaps you started yoga as a way to alleviate stress or anxiety, and now you find yourself feeling more centered and grounded in your daily life. Maybe you have noticed an improvement in your focus and concentration, or you have developed a greater sense of self-compassion and acceptance. These achievements, no matter how small they may seem, are worth celebrating.

Reflecting on your journey and achievements is not about comparing yourself to others or seeking external validation. It is about recognizing your own progress and growth on a personal level. Allow yourself to be proud of the steps you have taken, the obstacles you have overcome, and the positive changes you have experienced.

As you reflect on your journey, consider journaling your thoughts and feelings. Writing can be a powerful tool for self-expression and self-reflection. Take the time to explore your emotions, thoughts, and insights that have arisen throughout your yoga practice. By putting pen to paper, you can gain clarity and a deeper understanding of your journey.

Remember, this reflection is not meant to be a one-time exercise but an ongoing practice. As you continue on your yoga journey, it is important to periodically reflect on your progress, reassess your goals, and acknowledge your achievements. By doing so, you can cultivate a greater sense of gratitude, self-awareness, and overall mental well-being.

In conclusion, reflecting on your journey and achievements in yoga is a powerful practice that nurtures your mental health. Take the time to celebrate your progress, acknowledge your achievements, and embrace the transformative power of yoga in your life. By doing so, you can continue to grow, evolve, and experience the healing benefits of this ancient practice.

Acknowledging the Ongoing Nature of Mental Health and Self-Care

In the fast-paced and stressful world we live in, mental health has become a pressing issue for everyone. It affects people of all ages, genders, and backgrounds. Yoga, a practice that integrates physical movement, breath control, and mindfulness, has emerged as a powerful tool in nurturing mental health. This subchapter aims to shed light on the ongoing nature of mental health and the importance of self-care, with a specific focus on the niche of yoga.

One crucial aspect of mental health that often goes unnoticed is the fact that it is an ongoing journey. Mental health is not a destination that can be reached and forgotten about. It requires continuous attention and care, just like our physical health. Acknowledging this ongoing nature is the first step towards creating a sustainable mental health routine.

Yoga, with its holistic approach, provides a perfect platform for nurturing mental health. It encourages self-reflection, self-compassion, and self-awareness, all of which are essential for maintaining good mental health. By regularly practicing yoga, individuals can develop a deeper understanding of their own thoughts, emotions, and triggers. This awareness allows them to make conscious choices that positively impact their mental well-being.

Self-care is another crucial element of mental health that often gets neglected. All too often, we prioritize the needs of others and neglect our own well-being. Yoga teaches us to prioritize self-care and offers a multitude of practices that help us unwind, recharge, and reconnect with ourselves. Whether it's through gentle stretching, meditation, or deep breathing exercises, yoga provides numerous tools for self-care that can be easily incorporated into our daily lives.

Furthermore, practicing yoga in a supportive and inclusive community can significantly enhance mental health. The sense of belonging and connection that arises from practicing yoga with others fosters a sense of support and understanding. It reminds us that we are not alone in our struggles and that there are people who care and can offer guidance when needed.

In conclusion, mental health is an ongoing journey that requires continuous attention and self-care. Yoga provides a powerful framework for nurturing mental health by promoting self-awareness, self-compassion, and self-care. By integrating yoga into our lives, we can develop the tools and support necessary to maintain good mental health, benefiting not only ourselves but also those around us.

Inspiring Others to Discover the Transformative Benefits of Yoga

Yoga is a practice that has been revered for centuries, originating in ancient India. It is not just a physical exercise but a way of life that encompasses the mind, body, and spirit. The transformative benefits of yoga are vast and have the power to positively impact every aspect of our lives. In this subchapter, we delve into the importance of inspiring others to embrace yoga and unlock its healing potential.

Yoga is not limited to a specific age group, gender, or fitness level. It is a practice that can be adapted and personalized to suit everyone's needs. Whether you are a beginner or an advanced practitioner, yoga has something unique to offer. By sharing our own experiences and journeys with yoga, we can inspire others to embark on their own path of self-discovery and healing.

One of the most significant benefits of yoga is its ability to enhance mental health. In today's fast-paced and stressful world, anxiety, depression, and other mental health issues have become increasingly prevalent. Yoga provides a sanctuary for individuals to quiet their minds, find inner peace, and develop a deeper connection with themselves. By sharing stories of personal growth and mental well-being, we can encourage others to explore yoga as a powerful tool for nurturing their mental health.

Additionally, yoga offers numerous physical benefits. Regular practice can improve flexibility, strength, and posture. It can also alleviate chronic pain and enhance overall physical well-being. As we share our own physical transformations and the positive impact yoga has had on our bodies, we can motivate others to embrace the practice and experience these benefits for themselves.

Furthermore, yoga promotes a sense of community and connection. By practicing together, we can create a supportive environment that fosters growth and healing. Sharing stories of the profound connections we have formed through yoga can inspire others to seek out similar experiences and build a network of like-minded individuals.

In conclusion, inspiring others to discover the transformative benefits of yoga is a powerful endeavor. By sharing our personal stories, experiences, and the multitude of benefits yoga has to offer, we can ignite a spark within others to explore this ancient practice. Whether it be for mental health, physical well-being, or a sense of community, yoga has the potential to enrich and transform the lives of every individual who embraces it. Let us come together and inspire others to embark on their own journey of self-discovery and healing through the practice of yoga.